Going Gluten Free

A Quick Start Guide for a Gluten-Free Diet

by Jennifer Wells

2013 by United Publishing House

Going Gluten Free: A Quick Start Guide for a Gluten Free Diet

ISBN-13: 978-1492792819
ISBN-10: 1492792810

www.UnitedPublishingHouse.com
Email: Authors@UnitedPublishingHouse.com

Printed in U.S.A

Table of Contents

Other Books by Jennifer Wells

The Green Smoothie: A Quick Start Guide about Vegetable Smoothie for Good Health (eBook and print)

Juice for Health: Juice Fasting for Health and Wellness (eBook)

Top 10 Tips to Help You Lose Weight (eBook)

Gluten-Free Kids: A Quick Start Guide for a Healthy Kids Diet (eBook and audiobook)

A Quick Start Guide to Beginning Yoga (eBook)

Detox Solutions for Healthier Living (eBook)

The Hidden Secrets to Better Sleep (eBook)

Loving It Raw: Understanding the Raw Food Diet (eBook)

Introduction

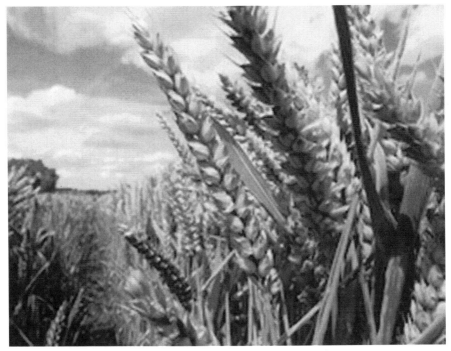

Over the last several years, there has been a great deal of public awareness and research done concerning the condition and symptoms of gluten sensitivity. Whether a person experiences mild bloating after eating products containing gluten or suffers severe cramping and headaches, those affected by gluten intolerance and Celiac Disease appear to be on the rise.

Come and spend some time with me as you learn:

- What gluten is

- How gluten free differs from grain free

- What happens when your body doesn't like gluten

- How to know if a product has gluten in it

- Discover strange places where gluten can "hide"

- Find helpful resources to further your investigation concerning Celiac Disease and gluten sensitivity

    This quick-start guide will give you an overview of how to begin to live a gluten-free lifestyle. It presents information you can process quickly. You will discover some of the basics involved in going gluten free so you will know which areas to tackle first, how to clean out your pantry and refrigerator, and what a shopping list looks like.

    If you suspect that you may be sensitive to gluten, think you cannot tolerate it, or you or someone you love have been diagnosed with Celiac Disease, then this resource will help you tremendously as you begin a lifestyle change of "Going Gluten Free."

What Is Gluten?

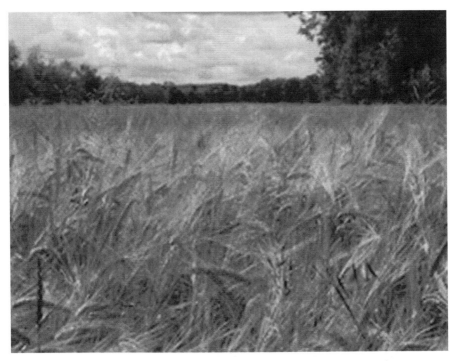

Although grains are classified as carbohydrates, about 10 to 15 per-cent of a kernel of grain is actually protein. The "germ" of the wheat that will become a new plant is mostly protein. The types of proteins vary from plant to plant, but in many grains, the most plentiful protein is gluten. In wheat, gluten makes up about 80% of the protein.

When water is added to flour made from ground-up wheat kernels, the mixture becomes an elastic, sticky, and gooey substance. It is the gluten within the dough ball that enables bread to rise and gives it its strength and texture.

Once kneading begins, the gluten causes long and flexible strands to develop in the dough. Then when yeast is added to the dough, these strands capture the gases released by the yeast, and the dough rises. As the dough cooks, it cements the strands of the gluten protein into place and allows the dough to remain in a solid, height-ened form.

Gluten is responsible for the chewiness of bread. Compare French baguettes with the softness and light airy texture of a cake. The differences in texture are determined by how much the gluten is developed. For chewiness, the gluten is kneaded extensively; for a cake, very little kneading or mixing is done. Yet, without gluten, foods like bagels, pizza, doughnuts and yeast breads would not exist as we know them today.

Gluten is found in grains like spelt, kamut, wheat, rye, graham, semolina, triticale, einkorn, durum, barley, farro, and bulgur wheat. Because flours like corn and rye have no gluten in them, wheat flour has to be added to them so loaves of bread can be made out of these flours. You see, without the gluten, yeast breads simply wouldn't get off the ground.

Oats normally do not contain gluten; however, oats that are processed commercially can easily become contaminated with gluten due to exposing this grain to other grains that do contain gluten. Great care and keeping grains separated during processing and storing have to occur in order to eliminate cross-contamination of gluten grains with non-gluten grains.

Now that you know a little bit more of what gluten is, in the next chapter I will discuss whether or not gluten is bad for you.

Is Gluten Bad for Me?

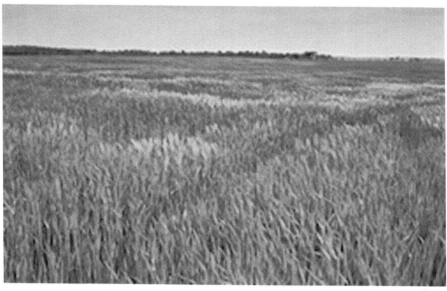

Although Celiac Disease was first described nearly two thousand years ago,(1) it has only been in the past few decades that the link between gluten and this chronic, debilitating disease has become clear. Celiac is an autoimmune disease, one of a class of diseases where your own immune system attacks normal cells within your body.

When a person has celiac disease, antibodies are formed against gliadin, a component protein of gluten. These antibodies attack the lining of the small intestine, damaging the small finger-like projections of these cells called "villi." With repeated damage, these villi become atrophic, and their ability to absorb nutrients is lessened. Along with this mal-absorption, the lining of the intestine also becomes "leaky," and toxic proteins that ordinarily could not enter the blood stream are able to pass through the intestinal wall and travel throughout the body.

Whenever someone with Celiac Disease – and to a lesser extent someone with gluten sensitivity – eats a product that has gluten in it, it triggers an autoimmune response. This attack can cause inflammation in many organ systems wherever the antibodies find similar proteins to attack. Because your body is literally fighting against itself, certain side effects result that you may not even realize are due to your gluten intake.

When this happens, here are some of the following symptoms that can occur:

- Fogginess
- Joint pain
- Headaches
- Abdominal pain
- Extremities becoming numb
- Diarrhea
- Bloating
- Fatigue
- Depression
- Fertility issues
- Eczema

As more research is being conducted in the area of Celiac Disease and gluten sensitivity, it has become apparent that gluten is turning out to be a real problem for many people—even for many who don't even realize it.

According to an article written by The American College of Gastroenterology cited on the Celiac Disease Foundation's website, *"Celiac disease prevalence is estimated to be near to 1:100 in Western countries. However, a much higher percentage of the general population than this 1% consider themselves to be suffering from wheat sensitivity and exclude wheat from their diet on the basis of their negative experience after eating wheat-containing foods."*[2] Although estimates vary widely, some believe as many as 1 in 3 people in our society may experience gluten sensitivity.

Other Reasons to Avoid Gluten

Even if you don't have a sensitivity to gluten, there may be other reasons to avoid it. (Note that some researchers suggest that you not discount the possibility of gluten sensitivity without eliminating gluten from your diet for a time).

Because gluten-containing grains are high in carbohydrates, this means insulin levels become elevated after you eat them. Whenever you eat, your blood sugar or glucose levels begin to rise. Ideally, you want blood glucose to rise slowly and maintain a fairly constant level – without fast rises that result in high peaks in sugar levels – followed by gently falling blood sugar levels that subtly warn you that you're hungry and it's time to eat again. You never want to suddenly feel famished or shaky.

All foods that affect your blood-sugar levels have been given a number on a scale called the Glycemic Index Foods List, determined scientifically by how your blood levels are affected. Foods that are low on the GI scale are ones like vegetables, nuts, and fruits. Foods that have a high GI score are foods like potatoes, rice, and breads. Surprisingly, even whole grain breads are at the high end of the scale.

Using this scale, eating pure glucose would have a glycemic index number of 100, which would cause a rapid rise in blood glucose and a high insulin response as well.

As a guide, foods are divided into three categories, depending upon how they affect your blood sugar levels:(3)

1. Low GI Foods – ranging from 0 to 55

2. Medium GI Foods – ranging from 56 to 70

3. High GI Foods – ranging from 70 to 100

To demonstrate how this works, here are a few grains and some grain products along with their corresponding number on the glycemic index:

- Bulgur wheat – 48
- Brown rice – 54
- Pita bread – 57
- Couscous – 65
- Whole wheat bread – 68
- Bagel – 72
- White bread – 79
- French bread – 95

As you can see, grains cause a rapid rise in blood sugar, as well as a strong insulin release. Amazingly, all of these bread products have a higher number on the scale than if you ate table sugar because sucrose only registers 50 on the GI scale. It isn't the gluten in bread causing the problems here, however. Decreasing gluten-containing foods in your diet will diminish the problems brought on with rapid changes in blood sugar.

A final problem associated with gluten-containing foods is the recently discovered fact that proteins within the gluten family can interact with the opiate receptors in your brain. You may have joked in the past that you were addicted to doughnuts, yet little did you know just how true this statement is! Not convinced? Think back to the last time you started a low-carb diet. You probably experienced "low-carb flu"—a period lasting several days early in your diet when you had to endure flu-like symptoms from carb withdrawal.

In his book, **The Paleo Solution,** author Robb Wolf humorously describes how hard it is to talk people into giving up gluten-filled grains from their diet:

"Not only do grains make you sick by raising insulin levels, messing up your fatty acid ratios and irritating your gut, but they are also addictive. Grains, particularly the gluten-containing grains, contain molecules that fit into the opiate receptors in our brain. You know, the same receptors that work with heroine, morphine, and Vicodin? Most people can take or leave stuff like corn tortillas and rice. [They don't contain gluten] Suggest that people should perhaps forgo bread and pasta for their health and they will bury a butter knife in your forehead before you can say "whole wheat!" (4)

The Best Test for Gluten Sensitivity

Still not completely sure gluten is a problem for you? Then try the advice of many who have gone before you:

1. Abstain from eating any gluten for 30 days and see how you feel at the end of the time period

2. At the end of 30 days, try eating something with gluten in it and see what happens and how it makes you feel

Like many who have done this, you may experience a complete disappearance of symptoms you thought you were destined to live with forever – symptoms like irritable bowel syndrome, eczema, headaches, and others listed above. However, when gluten is eliminated, something almost *magical* can happen: you may find yourself feeling better at the end of the 30 days than you ever thought possible. For the first time, your days are symptom-free.

If you suspect that you are experiencing problems with gluten as we've discussed here, consider the author's advice of The New York Times Bestseller, **Wheat Belly:** *"Treatment is simple: complete avoidance of anything containing gluten."* (5)

So, does all this mean that gluten could be a villain in your life? Well, try eliminating it and see!

Why Go Gluten Free?

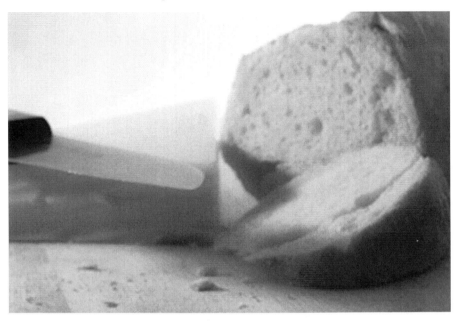

At this point, you may be thinking, "Okay. Thank you for telling me about gluten and what it can do. It sounds like some people have a tough time. But, I like my sandwich bread and I want my pizza crust chewy. I don't understand why anyone would want to go gluten free unless they had to."

Unfortunately, for all that gluten accomplishes in cooking, there are many people that become sick from eating it and even being exposed to it. Additionally, it is becoming clear that many more have varying degrees of gluten sensitivity and need to limit their intake of this protein.

Limiting your exposure and intake of gluten can be difficult at first because many foods contain small amounts of gluten and can create uncomfortable symptoms if you are sensitive to it.

Gluten is not only found in breads and pizzas, but it is also used in flavorings and thickeners in many foods. This is why learning to read labels carefully and what product ingredients contain gluten are so important when trying to avoid ingesting it.

Added to the task of reading labels, contamination of foods containing gluten often come in contact with non-gluten foods during the manufacturing process, resulting in gluten contaminating non-gluten foods. This is why it is so important to know how and where products are produced.

To begin to comprehend how difficult it can be to know if foods have gluten in them or not, here is a short list to consider. As you will see, gluten can be found in some of the strangest places. For instance, did you know that gluten can be found in:

- Licorice
- Flavored potato chips
- Soy sauce
- Chicken and beef broths
- Teas like holiday and specialty flavors
- Beer
- Dressings
- Marinades and
- Soups

And here are some others that could be included in the list:

- Orzo
- Panko
- Strudel
- Matzo
- Croutons
- Barley
- Bran

- Bulgur

- Rye

- Graham flour

- Durum

- Farina

- Modified food starch

- Burrito

- Couscous

- Semolina

This is by no means an exhaustive list! Those who have Celiac Disease, or those who are gluten intolerant, have a huge job of learning what foods they can eat and those they must avoid. Fortunately, more and more information is becoming available as manufacturers and consumers find it necessary to address this issue. Products are being created that are labeled "gluten free" as a way of helping consumers discover products that are safe for their dietary needs.

As more and more research is being done concerning foods and how they affect our bodies, gluten is being eliminated in the diets of those not only gluten-sensitive, gluten-intolerant, or those who have Celiac Disease, but this form of eating is gaining popularity with people who don't appear to have a noticeable problem eating it. Eliminating gluten is becoming a choice many people are making in an effort to cut carbs and lose weight.

In the next chapter, I am going to share with you some differences between a gluten-free diet and a grain-free one.

How Does Gluten Free Compare to Grain Free?

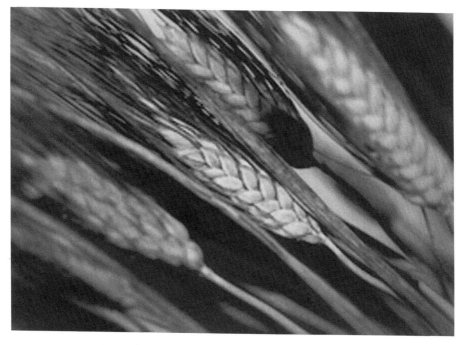

Simply put, gluten free means the gluten protein is not present in any product. Grain free, however, means just that –*no grains allowed!* If you were to decide to go grain free, this means you would no longer eat any kind of grain – no wheat, rice, corn, barley – none!

While gluten is found in some grains, it is not in others. This means if you are going to go "gluten free," it is possible to still enjoy *some* grains but you need to learn which ones don't contain gluten. Some examples of grains without gluten are rice, buckwheat, teff, corn, and oat.

Grains such as spelt, wheat, kamut, rye, and barley are grains that do have gluten – some higher than others, but they all contain certain percentages of gluten. That's why people who choose to go gluten-free can still eat grains, whereas people who go grain-free choose to eliminate them all together. Some reasons why people commonly choose to eliminate grains totally from their diet is because they want to cut carbs, they want to lose weight, or they discover they are sensitive to gluten. This way of eating is often known as a Paleo diet, a Primal diet, the Caveman diet, and a Paleolithic diet just to name a few.

As you can imagine, Paleolithic-diet eaters often experience signs of improved health because not only have they given up a huge percentage of carbohydrates – which are also high on the glycemic index – but they often notice symptoms they had related to gluten intolerance begin to disappear, often without realizing their disappearance was possible.

When someone decides to eliminate gluten from their diet, they can continue to enjoy grains like oat, buckwheat, rice, and sorghum. Since these grains do not contain gluten, they have to be used in different combinations with other flours and ingredients in order to achieve breads, pastas, and pizza crusts similar to gluten products.

If you find it necessary to eliminate gluten from your diet, or you desire to, here is an important note before we leave this section. Whenever you see, "wheat-free" on food labels, realize this does NOT necessarily mean "gluten-free." If barley or rye is used in place of a wheat ingredient, it does not mean it is gluten-free because both barley and rye have gluten in them. Just one reason why going gluten-free takes some studying.

As you become better at label reading, you will discover that gluten hides in some very unique places and this is the topic we will discuss in the next chapter.

What Are Some Hidden Sources of Gluten?

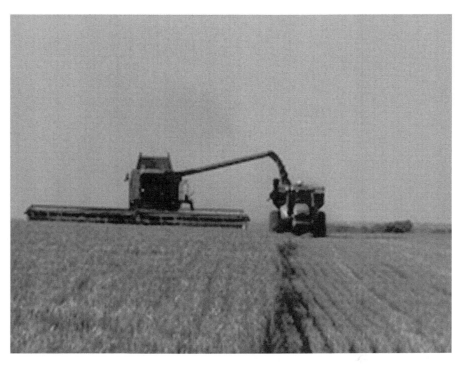

When you begin to become familiar with the names for wheat and its derivatives, you will begin to notice that gluten is not only in many of the foods we eat, but it can also be found in many non-food products as well. Here are some unusual places where gluten has been known to hide: (6)

- Cosmetics
- Lotions
- The glue on envelopes
- Powdered gloves
- Art supplies
- Paints
- Wallpaper paste
- Clay

- Play dough
- Lipstick
- Toothpaste
- Soaps
- Shampoos
- Mouthwash
- Detergents
- Bar soaps
- Sunscreen
- Medications

Along with some of the hidden sources of gluten in non-food products, you will notice strange names listed as ingredients on many food products containing gluten. Here is an incomplete list of ingredients that contain wheat. This list demonstrates that eliminating gluten from your diet will take time, education, and patience.

- Vitamin E processed from wheat germ
- Textured vegetable protein, also known as TVP
- Modified food starch when a product is made outside the US
- Maltodextrin
- Vegetable gums
- Mono & diglycerides
- Stabilizers
- Binders
- Fillers (7)

As you can see, you have to be on your guard when it comes to buying any processed foods. It will require learning the names and terms of ingredients containing gluten, as well as becoming familiar with companies that manufacture safe products that are gluten free.

While there are some companies that start making products considered gluten free, some may decide to change their methods of processing foods and begin to include wheat flours. This is just one reason why you will always need to read the packaging carefully and call the manufacturers anytime you are in doubt.

I realize there is a great deal of information to process when starting to adapt a gluten-free lifestyle, so in the next chapter, I'm going to walk you through ways to begin to make this change.

How Do I Begin a Gluten Free Lifestyle?

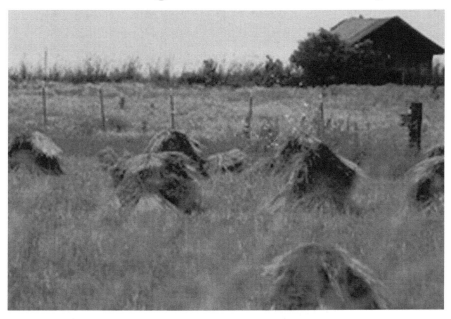

If you decide to eliminate gluten from your diet as well as your household, it can be quite confusing and time consuming; however, there are some main areas you can focus on first as you begin to make some decisions concerning how to change the way you eat.

Let's begin by taking some of the main categories of foods and break them down into manageable pieces. Let's begin with bread because this is one of the biggest changes you will have to make.

1. Grains and Breads: Bread is something you can continue to eat, ***however, it must be gluten-free bread.*** Realize that gluten-free breads can be made at home and are available for purchase, but the texture of these breads is definitely different from what you are used to with traditional breads. These breads can smell and even taste different. Their texture will take some getting used to. Give yourself time to get used to the newness of these types of breads and be patient with yourself.

There are numerous gluten-free breads on the market that can be purchased at bigger grocery chains and specialty grocery stores.

Start by checking the freezer section first. These breads are often frozen so their shelf life can be extended. Like many other products, some of them are good while others taste like sawdust. You will just have to experiment to see which ones you enjoy. Fortunately, new breads are being offered for sale all the time as manufacturers produce new combinations.

The other place to check is for recipes on the Internet. More and more people have begun to share their recipe efforts with others as they work together to find "enjoyable alternatives" to whole-grain breads.

In the meantime, consider using foods like lettuce, corn and brown rice tortillas for your sandwiches. These will give you options while you continue your search for a new type of sandwich bread.

Rice is gluten free. Whole grain brown rice is good, as well as risotto, basmati, and jasmine.

A special note about oats: You must be careful when buying oats. Even though oats do not contain gluten, if they are processed commercially, you must know if there is any chance of cross contamination especially during harvesting, storing and milling. If oats are processed with other grains that contain gluten, do not risk it. There are manufacturers that produce oats that are certified gluten-free. Go with these to play it safe and always look for gluten-free on the label.

2. Fruits and vegetables: Fortunately, all fruits and vegetables are gluten free when eaten fresh. When you buy them in cans or frozen, be sure to read the labels for any that may contain sauces and other additives. In the beginning, keep it simple and try to stay with fresh as much as possible.

3. Meats, Poultry, and Seafood: Red meats, pork, poultry, fish, and seafood are naturally gluten-free. The problems arise when sauces, broths, seasonings and marinades are added to them. Whenever possible, eat fresh or plain frozen meats so you know what you are consuming.

4. Dairy has two different aspects to it:

a.) To begin with, if you don't have any problems with dairy, then this area won't require very many changes. Consider cultured plain organic yogurts instead of flavored ones, then add your own honey and gluten-free fruit jams if you wish. Be aware that flavored yogurts may contain ingredients made with barley and added granolas so these can be a problem, too.

Aged cheeses are safest because the lactose levels are almost zero. As cheese ages, the lactose levels drop so even if you have some dairy issues, these are some of the safest ones to consume. Just make sure to watch for any added flavorings in the cheeses you eat.

If you choose to eat low-fat dairy foods, be sure to watch for any fillers and added starches. Some of these may prove to have gluten in them. Consider gluten-free vegan cheese alternatives that are made from almonds and rice. Start with labels that say "gluten-free" on the packaging and go from there. Call the manufacturers if you have any questions and be sure you learn the derivative names for casein, whey and lactose.

b.) The second part of the dairy issue concerns gluten-sensitive people that may also have problems with the casein and whey proteins in milk, as well as milk sugar called lactose. If you find you still have symptoms after eliminating gluten from your diet, consider eliminating dairy for a time to see if your symptoms disappear. Many experts recommend a period of 30 days. If this proves to be your situation, you will need to take added measures to eliminate milk proteins and lactose from your diet.

5. Miscellaneous Foods:

- Most **tofu** is gluten-free. Read labels carefully and watch out for versions that contain flavorings

- **Seitan** is made from vital wheat gluten and must be avoided

- **Potatoes** are all gluten free. If you buy them processed, read the labels for any additives like sauces or flavorings

- **Polenta** is made from cornmeal and should say "gluten free" on the packaging to ensure its safety

Foods to Avoid

When striving to eat a gluten-free diet, it is helpful to consider numerous other foods. Because your intestines have been inflamed and damaged over time, there are some things to do, and avoid, as you find your way to recovery.

1. Avoid processed foods, junk food, fast food, and pre-packaged snack foods as much as possible. It is easy for food to become cross-contaminated in restaurants and packaging plants unless they are totally dedicated to being gluten free

2. Be sure and read the labels on **herbal teas and tea blends.** Some of these drinks have flavors and additives that contain malt and barley

3. Sugar alcohols can negatively affect your digestive system by causing bloating, gas pains, and even diarrhea so avoid products that contain these. Try to eat organic and raw sugars that are not highly processed

4. Beer is to be avoided unless you can find one that says it is gluten-free

As you can see, beginning a lifestyle of eating and living gluten free is a big undertaking, but one that can be accomplished one food group at a time. While this is certainly not an exhaustive list, it is *very important* to learn terminology and the derivative names for wheat.

Now let's start to see what some meals and snack ideas will look like. I think you will be pleased with the number of options available to you.

What Do Meals and Snacks Look Like?

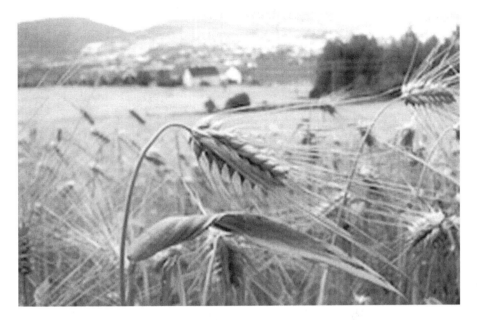

As you begin to wrap your mind around what it means to live gluten-free, I thought it would be helpful to give you some practical ideas of what snacks and mealtimes can look like. There are many foods available to you and this chapter is meant to help get your creative juices flowing while you become comfortable with label reading and food preparation.

You can find other ideas and resources on the Internet as more and more people are sharing their experiences and food choices found in the marketplace.

Snack Ideas

- Apple slices with a chunk of aged cheddar cheese
- Salads with almonds, pecans, or walnuts added
- Try some fresh grapes with aged cheddar cheese

- Make your own flavored yogurt using plain cultured organic yogurt and natural preserves. Strive for preserves labeled low sugar or no sugar added

- Bananas and fresh-ground peanut butter on a corn tortilla

- Try baby carrots or sticks dipped in your favorite salsa or gluten-free dip. Consider making your own dips as well

- Make your own trail mix with dried apples, raisins, and nuts

- Look for gluten-free corn tortilla chips and enjoy your favorite salsa or homemade guacamole dip

- Rice cakes are good with natural nut butters. Add raw honey if you like

- There are gluten-free goodies you can buy like ice cream and sorbets, popsicles and fruit bars. Baked goods are available for purchase as well

Mealtime Ideas

- Stir-fry is a great way to eat healthy and gluten-free. Cut up a bunch of fresh vegetables or use frozen vegetables without added flavorings and sauces. Add in some meat strips like beef or chicken, and top with gluten-free sauces

- Have a baked potato night. Cook up whole white or sweet potatoes and enjoy adding vegetables, homemade meat sauces and chilies that you know are gluten-free, then sprinkle on some aged shredded cheeses

- Soups and stews for lunch and dinner are great choices. Meats, natural broths, and vegetables are delicious

- Use rice with your stir-fry and sauces

- Lunches can be similar to dinners with salads containing meat strips, nuts, dried and fresh fruits

- Leftovers from last night's dinner are always good, too
- Breakfast time gives possibilities for egg dishes like frittatas that contain onions, mushrooms, bell peppers and aged cheeses
- Look for cereals that are labeled "gluten-free" and enjoy with almond or rice milk. Be sure to read labels to make sure they are gluten free
- Gluten-free waffles are readily available on the market now. Top with fresh fruit or pure maple syrup
- Quinoa, millet, and rice can be cooked to make a hearty breakfast cereal topped with cinnamon, raw honey or pure maple syrup and nuts
- Smoothies made with plain cultured yogurt, frozen fruits and honey make a great breakfast or dessert

Remember, all vegetables and fruits are gluten free, as are meats, poultry, pork, fish and seafood - as long as they haven't been processed with added sauces and flavorings that contain gluten products.

As you become more confident in your learning, use some of these meal ideas, and when your creativity kicks in, you will see that you have probably been eating a great deal of foods that were gluten-free but you did not realize it. Now that you are starting to see what you are allowed to eat and what must be avoided, it is time to tackle your pantry, refrigerator and freezer.

What Will My Pantry and Refrigerator Look Like?

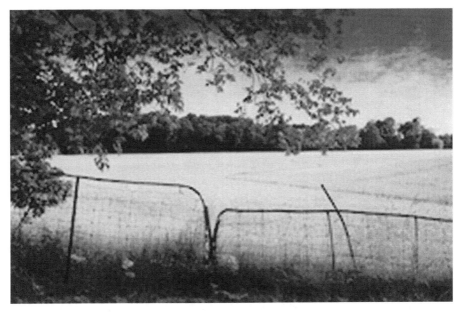

Once you decide you want, or need to go gluten free, you will have to tackle the foods you already have in your home. This requires reading labels on all the items in your refrigerator, freezer and pantry cabinets.

As you begin, if any of the items contain gluten and they are unopened, consider giving the items to friends who can eat gluten, your local food bank or other charitable organizations. If items are already opened, empty the contents and recycle the container if this is a service available in your area.

Some items are ones you won't be sure about because you may not have had time to research whether or not products with added ingredients contain gluten. In this case, put them aside so you can look them up and have your questions answered.

For some that have severe cases of gluten sensitivity or Celiac Disease, it may be necessary to remove old cutting boards, repaint your walls, clean handles and knobs, and wipe down countertops with disinfectants. Vacuuming, wiping, scrubbing, and scraping can be quite laborious in the beginning, but once these things are accomplished, life can begin to get back to some form of routine for you.

In all of your changes and preparations, give yourself time! It's a huge task to go through everything you have stored in your refrigerator, freezer and cabinets and decontaminate your working space, but these are things to take in stride and accomplish one at a time.

Once you've tackled your supply of food and decided which ones should be kept and which ones should be eliminated, you'll probably need to go grocery shopping. In the next section, I will walk you through what a shopping trip might look like.

What Do I Buy at the Grocery Store?

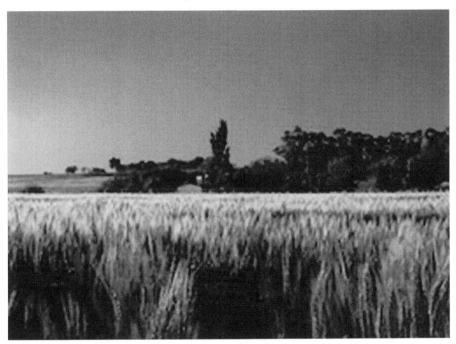

Your first trip to the grocery store can be overwhelming. Reading labels and the fine print on packaging can take hours.

Before you tackle the store though, consider coming up with a plan that will work for you. You will need to develop your own personal strategy. As you've worked your way through the information presented here so far, you have seen ideas for snacks and mealtimes, as well as foods to avoid and ones to try.

A good place to begin is to start with your normal menu plans and substitute ingredients and products with ones you know to be gluten free.

Next, take a good look at some of the items I will share with you and decide which ones work for you and your family. Pick out items you are familiar with and ones that are considered safe and make your own personalized shopping list.

Another tip would be to write down brand names you've read about on the Internet or have learned about from magazines, books and friends that have been shown to be gluten free and seem to interest you.

As you transition over to a gluten-free diet, one of the first places to make changes is going to be concerning grains. Eliminate the ones you have learned that have gluten in them and become familiar with the alternatives available to you. Below I have listed some gluten-free grains and flours you can eat and use in your cooking.

When you buy various flours and nut meals, try to purchase products with labels that say "organic, gluten-free, whole grain, and all-natural."

1. Millet flour: You can buy millet seeds and make flour using a high-speed blender. It's a good source of protein, B-complex, lecithin, magnesium, and potassium.

2. Brown rice flour: This whole grain is used a great deal to replace wheat flour and is often used as part of a gluten-free, all-purpose baking mix. It is high in protein, fiber, and B vitamins.

3. Sweet rice flour: This is a nice addition to baking mixes used for breads and pizzas.

4. Amaranth flour: This is often used in combination with other flours for baking. It is high in protein, fiber, zinc, calcium and iron.

5. Sorghum flour: Often used in recipes to replace wheat flour, it adds a great texture to baked goods. It is high in antioxidants, fiber, iron, and protein.

6. Quinoa flour and flakes: This grain is often used in recipes for making muffins, breads, and cookies. A complete protein containing calcium, fiber, manganese, copper, and magnesium and gives baked goods a nutty taste. Some people enjoy substituting quinoa for oatmeal.

7. Buckwheat flour and groats: A nutritious grain with a distinctive flavor often used in soups, cereals, waffles, and pancakes.

High in fiber, B vitamins and lysine, it is also rich in other vitamins like copper, iron, magnesium, and manganese.

8. Teff flour: A grain high in nutrients, it contains iron, calcium, vitamin C, fiber and thiamin and adds moistness to baked goods.

9. Almond flour and almond meal: A flour made from almonds that is highly nutritious, easy to find and use. It is low in carbs and sugars, but high in protein and often used for crusts.

10. Coconut flour: Flour made from the meat of the coconut, it has many nutrients, is a great source of fiber, and adds moisture to baked goods.

11. Corn flour and corn meal: Corn flour is ground finer than corn meal. Look for the words "whole" and "not degermed" to ensure it hasn't been genetically modified. Rich in fiber and antioxidants, corn meal and flour adds a nutty taste to baked goods.

12. Oat flour: Flour that is high in minerals and fiber, be sure to look for labeling that promises no cross-contamination with other grains.

Because of the nature of these flours and the fact that they don't contain any gluten, they have to be used in combinations with other flours for creating most baked goods. There are increasingly more helpful resources and cookbooks coming out on the market that can help you with this type of cooking.

Fortunately, many items that you probably already eat are ones that don't have any gluten in them so it may not be as difficult for you to begin eating gluten free as you may have initially thought.

Nowadays, many products that are processed and labeled "gluten free" help make shopping easier for you. However, if you aren't sure or familiar with particular products, be sure to read the product's label carefully before purchasing it. In addition, contact the manufacturer to see if a product is processed in a plant where cross contamination occurs. There is often a phone number listed on the product you can call to make sure the product is safe for you. If it is not or you are not sure, do not buy it.

In this section, I want to provide you with some items for your shopping list that have been shown to be safe and gluten-free. If you would like a list of them so you can print them out and take the list to the grocery store, you will find a PDF file at UnitedPublishingHouse. com listed under the title of this book.

For the sake of time and space, I will give you a few examples from each of the main food categories. For a more thorough listing, once again the PDF can be found at UnitedPublishingHouse.com. (http://unitedpublishinghouse.com/going-gluten-free-a-quick-start-guide-for-a-gluten-free-diet/) (8)

A Gluten-Free Shopping List

Under the category of grains, pastas, cereals, and chips, the following are gluten-free and safe to purchase:

- Arrowroot starch

- Crackers made from corn, lentils, and brown rice varieties but make sure they are labeled gluten free

- Dry cereal varieties made with corn, rice, amaranth, millet, buckwheat, and soy

- Pastas made from brown rice, corn, peas, beans, potatoes, lentils, soy, or quinoa

- Plain corn chips

- Popcorn. Air-popped popcorn varieties and packages labeled gluten-free are best

- Rice varieties that are wild, brown, basmati, and risotto

- Rice cakes that are plain are the safest

- Taco shells made from corn
- Tortilla chips that are plain are safest

Under the category of dairy, here are some guidelines to follow: The low-fat varieties and the reduced fat cheeses are good to start with.

- Aged cheeses are best if you suspect dairy is an issue
- Cottage cheeses
- Cream cheeses
- When considering ice cream, be sure to read the labels for each flavor
- Milk
- Milk alternatives such as rice, soy, and almond
- Plain yogurts
- Sour creams

When it comes to buying fruits:

- All fresh fruits are gluten free. If you buy frozen fruits, be sure to check the label for any added ingredients

When purchasing vegetables and legumes:

- All fresh vegetables and frozen vegetables that do not have any added breading, additives, or sauces are safe. Be sure to read the packaging before buying any
- Canned beans are gluten-free
- All fresh varieties of potatoes are gluten-free. If buying canned or frozen, be sure to read the labels

In the category of meats, poultry, seafood and other proteins:

- All fresh meats, poultry, shellfish, and fish are gluten-free. If buying frozen or canned, be sure to check for additives such as breading

- Eggs are fine

- Plain tofu is best. Read labels if you wish to purchase flavored tofu

For the category of nuts and seeds:

- All nuts, nut butters, and seeds are fine

If using oils:

- Purchase coconut oil, olive oil, and nut oils

In the category of vinegars:

- Purchase apple cider, red wine, white wine, white, or balsamic

With herbs and spices:

- All pure herbs and spices are gluten-free. If you want to purchase herb and spice mixes, be sure to read the labels

In the area of baking goods and condiments, there are many to choose from. Some you are certainly familiar with like:

- Baking chocolate

- Baking powder

- Baking soda

- Cocoa powder

- Instant and ground coffees are fine. Be sure to check the ingredients of flavored coffees

- Extracts like vanilla, rum, and almond

- Garlic

- Honey

- Ketchup

- Mustard

- Pickles

- Salsa

- Sugar

- Black and green teas. Be sure to read the labels on flavored teas

When desiring to use sweeteners, focus on natural sugars like

- Raw honey

- Blackstrap molasses

- Pure maple syrup

From a health standpoint, try to eat the freshest and purest products you can afford. However, whenever you buy packaged or processed foods, be sure to read the labeling, which I know can be quite confusing.

To close out this section on grocery shopping, I want to share with you a list of additives that gluten-free. Although I am only going to share a few with you here, once again you can consult the PDF for a gluten-free shopping list at UnitedPublishingHouse.com

- Arrowroot

- Ascorbic acid

- Aspic

- BHA

- BTA

- Dextrose

- Fructose

- Guar gum

- Locust bean gum

- Malic acid

- Pectin

- Pepsin

- Sulfites

- Tapioca starch and flour

- Whey

- Xanthan gum

As you become familiar with items to buy and ones that are safe to eat, eventually you will find yourself wanting to eat out in restaurants or you need to grab a quick bite to eat.

In the next chapter, I will share with you some important guidelines to follow and questions to ask when you find yourself not being able to eat at home.

How Do I Eat Out and Remain Gluten Free?

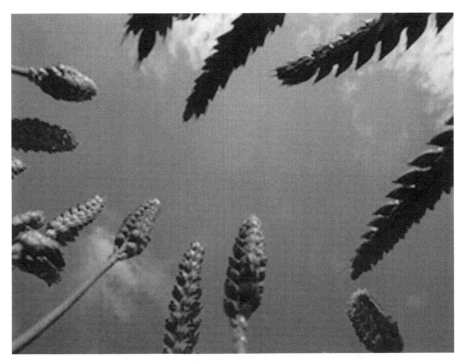

Initially, you may feel as though it is safest to always eat at home, and when you are first making changes in your diet, this may prove to be best. Give yourself time to learn what you are looking for and the questions you will need to ask when eating out.

As more and more people become aware of gluten-free eating and as restaurant chains strive to serve the public, eating out is becoming easier. However, there are still definite challenges involved if you are living a gluten-free lifestyle.

For starters, there are numerous regional and national restaurant chains that have started offering gluten-free menu items, as well as some fast-food chains. Knowing what to look for and how to ask questions are a big part of you feeling safe, remaining healthy and enjoying your dining experience.

The following list is helpful for equipping you when you are ready to venture out:

1. Choose your restaurant of choice wisely. Start by choosing restaurants that offer gluten-free entrées. Once you find some, you can ask questions of the manager and specifically the chef because they will have had training concerning this issue. While you may be tempted to question the server, they usually are not as familiar with food preparations as the manager and chef.

2. Check with the restaurant to see if they have a dedicated fryer for gluten-free frying. If you want fried foods, be sure to ask this question. Potatoes that are fried in the same fryer as battered onion rings are going to give you problems with gluten.

3. If desiring to order from the grill, check to see if marinades with gluten have been used on it. Gluten is often used in marinades for flavoring and thickening, so check with the manager to see if this will affect the item you want to order.

4. There can be a real problem with cross-contamination. For example, according to Chef Egan, *"Flour particles take three days to settle. If a kitchen is making their own bread or dough and it is a shared kitchen, then it's more of a challenge. Not many kitchens have a separate pastry kitchen."*(9)

5. When in doubt, ask questions. When ordering, be sure to ask how your food will be prepared to eliminate possibilities of cross contamination. Be sure you are satisfied with how your food will be prepared. When your food comes, oftentimes the manager will accompany your order; however, if not, be sure to ask the server questions of how it was prepared and to make sure it is exactly what you

ordered and how you ordered it. Ultimately, if you are not satisfied with the results, don't eat it.

Although it may prove awkward to receive your meal but not eat it, it is certainly better to go hungry for a little while rather than suffer the consequences of a meal gone awry.

Learning to feel confident about eating out may take you some time. Ask a friend to accompany you who is familiar with gluten-free cooking. Having two sets of ears and two people thinking along the same wavelength can diminish a lot of the stress involved in learning how to eat out successfully and enjoyably when first starting out.

In Closing

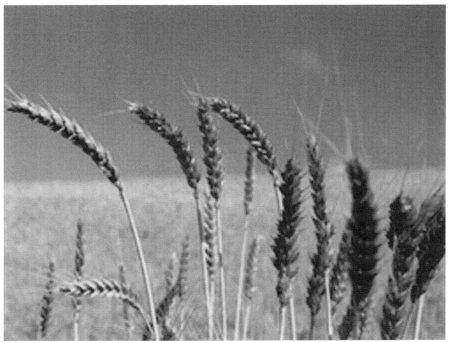

Whether you choose to eat gluten free, or have to because of intolerance or Celiac Disease, eating and living gluten free eventually becomes a way of life. Any time something as big as changing the way you eat, how you shop, products you use and how you live your life is going to take time.

One of the biggest challenges in living gluten free is giving yourself the time necessary to get educated about foods that contain gluten, what non-food products contain gluten, what needs to change in your home to keep gluten from re-entering, and how to enjoy dining out.

In addition, be aware that you will experience many different emotions as you make this transition. For example:

- Sometimes you will find yourself feeling sad as you begin to understand what eating gluten-free really means. There may even be a sense of mourning as you start to realize you won't be able to eat some of your favorite foods anymore because they contain gluten

- There will be times when you feel happy and relieved that you finally have a diagnosis because it helps to explain why you have been feeling the way you have

- Sometimes you will feel frustrated because things are more complicated and not as convenient as they were before

- Finally, realize you will experience these emotions off and on for the rest of your life. Accept that these emotions will affect you from time to time and try to determine what caused various emotions to occur so you can better handle them the next time

As you've discovered, there are many layers to this issue. Consider finding a support group online or one locally you can lean on to gain understanding and help.

While there is much to learn in the beginning, consider this lifestyle change like a new adventure; one that offers new chances to learn, opportunities for changes, and the ultimate goal – a chance for you to feel better than you ever have!

If you have been suffering from gluten related symptoms and you are finally on the road to eliminating them from your diet and life, you will begin to feel:

- More energetic

- Experience your fogginess lifting

- Be able to focus better for longer periods of time

- And have a much better outlook on life

And I'm sure you will agree—these are things worth striving for!

Where Can I Find More Information?

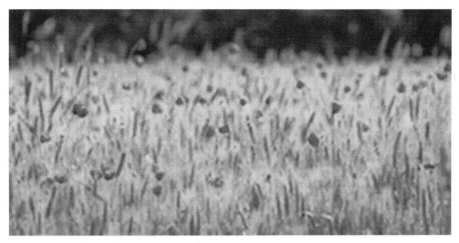

I have listed a few resources in this section that I believe you will find helpful during your search to discover more about a gluten-free lifestyle and to help you find support from others who are dealing with the same lifestyle changes as you.

Organizations you could research are:

1. *Celiac Disease and Gluten-Free Diet Information* (http://www.celiac.com/)

2. *National Foundation for Celiac Awareness* (http://www.celiaccentral.org/)

3. *The Great Life: Gluten-Free Updates from Celiac Central* (http://blog.vitacost.com/the-great-life/)

4. *Celiac Sprue Association: Celiacs Helping Celiacs* (http://www.csaceliacs.info/)

5. *Celiac Disease Awareness Campaign* (http://celiac.nih.gov/organizations.aspx)

6. *Celiac Support Groups: Organizations and Online Communities for People with Celiac Disease* (http://celiacdisease.about.com/od/theglutenfreediet/a/glutenfreeorgs.htm)

Some Celiac and Gluten-Free Bloggers are:

1. *Adventures of a Gluten Free Mom* (http://www.adventuresofa-glutenfreemom.com/)

2. *Gluten Free School: Gluten Free Learning Without Borders* (http://www.glutenfreeschool.com/)

3. *Gluten Free for Good: The Art & Science of Healthy Living* (http://www.glutenfreeforgood.com/blog/)

4. *No Gluten, No Problem* (http://noglutennoproblem.blogspot.com/)

5. *Manifest Vegan: Gluten-free, Animal Friendly Recipes* (http://www.allysonkramer.com/)

6. *Celiac and Gluten-free Bloggers* (http://www.celiaccentral.org/Resources/Gluten-Free-Bloggers/125/) This webpage offers many more choices for you to follow others who are on this adventure with you.

Other Books by Jennifer Wells

The Green Smoothie: A Quick Start Guide about Vegetable Smoothie for Good Health (eBook and print)

Juice for Health: Juice Fasting for Health and Wellness (eBook)

Top 10 Tips to Help You Lose Weight (eBook)

Gluten-Free Kids: A Quick Start Guide for a Healthy Kids Diet (eBook and audiobook)

A Quick Start Guide to Beginning Yoga (eBook)

Detox Solutions for Healthier Living (eBook)

The Hidden Secrets to Better Sleep (eBook)

Loving It Raw: Understanding the Raw Food Diet (eBook)

Acknowledgements

I would like to personally thank the following photographers for their creativity which can be found at *Flickr.com*.

- *Jams_123*
- *Rosa Dik 009 -- on & off*
- *Olgierd Pstrykotwórca*
- *loco's photos*
- *juzsan*
- *Cyron*
- *Aunt Owwee*
- *jon gos*
- *Robb North*
- *.:elNico:.*
- *marfis75*
- *Venex_jpb*
- *kaibara87*

About the Author

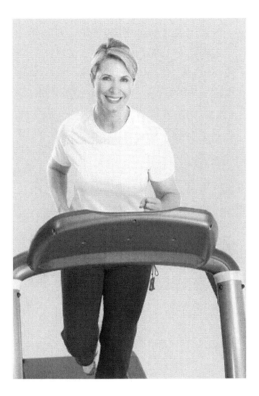

Always into sports and very active growing up, Jennifer never gave much thought to diet and exercise. Weight gain was not much of an issue. Then, after marriage and the birth of her twin boys, Jennifer noticed she had problems keeping her weight under control.

After numerous years of frustration, trying to get rid of stubborn pounds and not feeling as well as she wanted, Jennifer began her own personal research into diet and exercise. As a result, she ended up going back to school to get a degree in nutritional science.

Now she enjoys living a healthy lifestyle, spending time outdoors, teaching classes on nutrition at her local high school, and sharing healthy tips and information with family and friends.

And just in case you are curious, Jennifer is now back down to her weight before she had her four children.

Footnotes

1. "Coeliac Disease." Viewed online at http://en.wikipedia.org/wiki/Coeliac_disease on 09.12.12.

2. *The American Journal of Gastroenterology,* "Non-Celiac Wheat Sensitivity Diagnosed by Double-Blind Placebo-Controlled Challenge: Exploring a New Clinical Entity," August 29, 2012. Viewed online at www.celiac.org/images/stories/PDF/2012-08-29.pdf on 09.08.12.

3. Glycemic Index List of Foods. Viewed online at http://www.lowgi-health.com.au/category/what-is-glycemic-index/ on 09.08.12.

4. Robb Wolf, *The Paleo Solution Diet* (Las Vegas, NV: Victory Belt Publishing, 2010), 97.

5. William Davis, M.D., *Wheat Belly: Lose the Wheat, Lose the Weight, and Find Your Path Back to Health* (New York, NY: Rodale), 39-40.

6. "Hidden Sources of Gluten." Viewed online at http://www.celiac-solution.com/hidden-gluten.html on 09.12.12.

7. List from website listed in #1.

8. "The Ultimate Grocery List for Celiac Disease." Viewed online at http://www.joybauer.com/celiac/food-list.aspx on 09.07.12.

9. Kendall Egan, "How Restaurant Kitchens Really Work." *Gluten-Free Living,* Spring 2012, 43.

Made in the USA
San Bernardino, CA
05 January 2014